# WEIGHT LOSS BOOK FOR WOMEN

*How to Lose Weight and Feel Great: A Practical Guide for Busy Women"*

Jovita Michael

## Copyright © [2023], [Jovita Michael]

All rights reserved. No part of this book may be reproduced, stored, or transmitted by any means—whether auditory, graphic, mechanical, or electronic—without written permission of both the author and publisher, except in the case of brief excerpts used in critical articles and reviews.

This book is a work of non-fiction. The names, characters, places, and incidents are products of the author's imagination or have been used fictitiously. Any resemblance to actual persons, living or dead, events, or locales is entirely coincidental.

## TABLE OF CONTENT

INTRODUCTION ............................................................. 7

CHAPTER ONE ............................................................. 14

UNDERSTANDING YOUR WEIGHT LOSS GOAL ...................... 14

    Reflecting on your current lifestyle and health: ............... 15

    Set Realistic Goals: ........................................................ 16

    Create An Action Plan: .................................................. 18

    Track Your Progress: ..................................................... 19

    Reward Yourself: ........................................................... 20

CHAPTER TWO ............................................................. 22

UNDERSTANDING THE ROLE OF NUTRITION IN WEIGHT LOSS ............................................................................. 22

    EATING FOR WEIGHT LOSS ........................................ 25

    Lean Proteins: ............................................................... 26

    Fruits and Vegetables: ................................................... 26

    Whole Grains: ............................................................... 27

    Legumes: ....................................................................... 27

    Healthy Fats: ................................................................. 27

    HOW TO READ NUTRITION LABELS ......................... 28

    Serving Size: .................................................................. 28

    Calories: ......................................................................... 28

Nutrients: .................................................................................. 28

Percent Daily Value (%DV): ...................................................... 28

Ingredients: ............................................................................... 29

Check for Nutrient Claims: ...................................................... 29

CHAPTER THREE ........................................................................ 30

DESIGNING A WEIGHT LOSS MEAL PLAN ............................... 30

TIPS TO DESIGNING A WEIGHT LOSS MEAL PLAN FOR WOMEN ...................................................................................... 31

Consult with A Nutritionist or Dietitian: ................................. 31

Determine Your Calorie Needs: ............................................... 31

Plan Meals and Snacks. ............................................................ 32

Choose Nutrient-Dense Foods: ................................................ 32

Monitor Portion Sizes: .............................................................. 32

Stay Hydrated: ........................................................................... 33

Track Your Progress: ................................................................ 33

HOW TO COMBINE DIFFERENT TYPES OF MACRO NUTRIENTS TO OPTIMIZE WEIGHT LOSS FOR WOMEN .... 33

Carbohydrates: ........................................................................... 33

Fats: ............................................................................................ 34

Proteins: ..................................................................................... 34

MEAL PLAN TIME- TABLE FOR WEIGHT LOSS IN WOMEN ...................................................................................................... 35

ALTERNATIVE MEAL PLAN RECIPE WITH INGREDIENTS, INSTRUCTIONS AND PREP TIME ............ 40

CHAPTER FOUR ............ 72

MAKING HEALTHY EATING HABIT STICK FOR WEIGHT LOSS. ............ 72

- Prepare Meals Ahead Of Time: ............ 72
- Set Realistic Goals: ............ 73
- Make Healthy Swaps: ............ 73
- Track Your Progress: ............ 73
- Get Enough Sleep: ............ 74
- Stay Hydrated: ............ 74
- Move Your Body: ............ 74

CHAPTER FIVE ............ 75

AVOIDING COMMON DIET PITFALLS ............ 75

CHAPTER SIX ............ 78

INCORPORATING EXERCISE INTO YOUR WEIGHT LOSS PLAN ............ 78

- Start Small: ............ 79
- Make A Plan: ............ 80
- Find An Activity You Enjoy: ............ 80
- Set Goals: ............ 80
- Make Time for Yourself: ............ 80

Find an accountability partner: ........................................................... 81

TYPES OF EXERCISES FOR WEIGHT LOSS IN WOMEN ...... 81

CHAPTER SEVEN ................................................................................ 84

MAINTAINING YOUR WEIGHT LOSS ............................................ 84

Set Realistic Goals: ...................................................................... 85

Track Your Progress: ................................................................... 85

Eat Healthy: .................................................................................. 86

Exercise regularly: ....................................................................... 86

Stay Motivated: ............................................................................ 86

Manage Stress: ............................................................................. 87

Get Enough Sleep: ....................................................................... 87

Avoid Temptation: ....................................................................... 87

Be Consistent: .............................................................................. 87

CONCLUSION: .................................................................................... 89

# INTRODUCTION

Liz was an overweight woman who had been struggling with her weight for years. She had tried every diet and exercise program she could find, but nothing seemed to work. Finally, she decided to try something new - a **weight loss diet book for women.**

The book was full of helpful information about healthy eating, exercise habits and lifestyle changes. Liz took the advice to heart and began to make small changes in her life. She started to eat healthier foods and incorporated exercise into her daily routine. She also began to make an effort to stay away from sugary and processed foods.

After a few weeks of following the diet, Liz started to see results. She was losing weight and her energy levels were increasing. She felt more confident in her own skin and was happier than ever. Liz was so proud of her accomplishments that she decided to share her story with others. She posted her progress on social media and encouraged other women to pick up the book and create their own success stories.

As Liz's story spread, more and more women began to follow her lead. Liz was amazed at the response and realized that she had started something bigger than she ever expected.

Liz's story is an inspiring example of how making small changes can lead to big results.

She was able to create a healthier and happier life for herself by following the advice in the book. Her story has inspired countless other women to take the same steps and make their own success stories. Women have been struggling with weight loss for centuries. From dieting to intense exercise, women have tried it all in order to achieve their ideal weight. Unfortunately, many women are left feeling frustrated and overwhelmed by the sheer number of options available to them. This can lead to confusion and a sense of helplessness when it comes to achieving their desired weight loss goals.

The good news is that with the right plan and dedication, it is possible to lose weight and keep it off. It all starts with understanding how your body works and what you need to do in order to achieve your desired results. This includes developing a healthy diet and exercise plan and making lifestyle changes that will help you stay on track.

Weight loss for women can be a complicated process, but it doesn't have to be. By understanding the basics of nutrition and exercise, you can create a plan that works for your lifestyle and goals. This includes learning about how to choose healthy foods, how to plan meals, and how to incorporate physical activity into your daily routine. Additionally, making changes to your lifestyle such as reducing stress, getting adequate sleep, and managing your emotions can help to ensure that your weight loss journey is successful.

With the right combination of knowledge, dedication, and support, women can lose weight and keep it off. By taking the time to develop a plan that works for you and following it faithfully, you can reach your desired weight loss goals and live a healthier, more balanced life.

Weight loss is a common goal that many individuals strive for, and there are a variety of motivations that can drive an individual to make a change in their lifestyle. Exploring your motivations for weight loss can be an important part of creating a successful plan for achieving your goals.

One common motivation for weight loss is to improve overall health. Many people want to reduce their risk for chronic diseases, such as heart disease or diabetes, by losing weight. Additionally, having a healthy weight can help improve energy levels and reduce the risk of developing certain health conditions. Achieving a healthier body image is another common motivation for weight loss. Many individuals want to feel more confident and comfortable in their own skin. By setting realistic goals and creating healthy lifestyle habits, you can work towards feeling more confident in your own body.

Having a positive self-image can also be a motivating factor for weight loss. Feeling good about your body can provide you with a greater sense of self-esteem and self-worth.

Finally, another motivation for weight loss is to improve physical performance. Many athletes and fitness enthusiasts strive to achieve a certain level of performance or strength by improving their overall fitness.

No matter your motivation for weight loss, it is important to create a plan that is tailored to your needs and encourages healthy habits. Working with a healthcare professional can help you create a plan that is both safe and effective. Exploring your motivations for weight loss can be the key to creating a successful plan for reaching your goals.

# CHAPTER ONE

# UNDERSTANDING YOUR WEIGHT LOSS GOAL

Understanding your weight loss goals means having a clear idea of what you want to achieve, and what it will take to get there. It means having realistic expectations and understanding the importance of hard work and dedication. It means having a plan to achieve your goals and sticking to it. It means being aware of the potential obstacles you might encounter, and having strategies in place to overcome them. It also means being honest with yourself about how much you can realistically lose and how much effort it will take to get there. Finally, it means believing in yourself and having the confidence to reach your goals. This can be achieved by:

## Reflecting on your current lifestyle and health:

Reflecting on current lifestyle and health can be an important part of understanding and achieving weight loss goals. Taking an honest look at eating habits, physical activity levels, stress levels, and lifestyle choices can help to identify areas that need to be addressed in order to achieve the desired goals. Additionally, getting a better understanding of how these aspects of life affect the body and its ability to maintain a healthy weight can be helpful in creating a plan for success. Lastly, understanding potential barriers to success and how to overcome them can help to keep motivation high and provide the necessary guidance to reach the desired goals.

**Set Realistic Goals:** Setting realistic goals for weight loss involves understanding what is achievable, and setting achievable and sustainable targets. This means setting goals that are realistic in terms of both time and amount of weight lost. It is important to have both short-term goals and long-term goals. Short-term goals should be achievable and measurable, such as losing 1-2 pounds per week. Long-term goals should be more ambitious and can involve a larger amount of weight loss over a longer period of time.

When setting goals, it is important to break them down into manageable steps that do not overwhelm the individual. For example, a goal to lose 10 pounds in 2 weeks is not realistic and will likely lead to discouragement and frustration. Instead, an achievable goal could involve losing 1-2 pounds per week for a period of 5-10 weeks.

In addition to setting realistic goals, it is important to have realistic expectations for weight loss. Weight loss is a gradual process that requires patience and dedication. It is important to remember that no matter how hard someone works, it is not possible to achieve immediate results.

Finally, it is important to remember that weight loss is not only about the number on the scale. It is also about developing a healthy lifestyle that includes regular physical activity, healthy eating habits, and stress-relieving activities. These habits will help an individual reach their goals and maintain a healthy weight.

**Create An Action Plan:** An action plan for weight loss is a comprehensive strategy that outlines the steps needed to reach your desired weight loss goals. It should include small, attainable goals that are achievable in the short-term, as well as long-term goals.

The plan should also include a detailed diet and exercise program, along with a way to track your progress. The action plan should be tailored to your individual needs and should encompass all aspects of your lifestyle. Additionally, the action plan should also include ways to stay motivated, such as setting rewards for yourself and finding an accountability partner.

**Track Your Progress:** Tracking your progress for weight loss means keeping a record of your weight, diet, exercise and any other relevant information related to your weight loss goals. It involves keeping track of your overall weight and body measurements, such as your waist circumference, body fat percentage, and body mass index (BMI). You may also want to track your calorie intake and expenditure, food choices, and other lifestyle habits. Tracking your progress can help you identify any areas where you may need to make changes or adjustments to your diet and exercise regimen in order to reach your goals. It can also help you stay motivated and provide a sense of accomplishment as you watch your progress over time.

**Reward Yourself:** To reward yourself for weight loss means to celebrate your accomplishment by doing something special that is meaningful to you. This could be anything from a shopping spree, a massage, a day at the spa, a fancy dinner, or a weekend getaway. The reward should be meaningful and motivating, and something that you can look forward to as an incentive to continue working towards your weight loss goals.

# CHAPTER TWO

# UNDERSTANDING THE ROLE OF NUTRITION IN WEIGHT LOSS

Understanding the role of nutrition in weight loss is essential for those looking to achieve and maintain a healthy weight. Nutrition plays a key role in weight loss, as it not only helps to provide the body with the fuel it needs to function, but also helps to keep hunger and cravings at bay. Proper nutrition also helps to ensure that the body is receiving the essential vitamins and minerals it needs to stay healthy. Eating a balanced diet that is rich in lean proteins, whole grains, fresh fruits and vegetables, and healthy fats can help to control hunger, boost metabolism, and provide the body with the nutrients it needs to stay healthy and empowered. Additionally, avoiding processed foods, sugary snacks, and high-calorie beverages can help to reduce the number of empty calories consumed, and promote weight loss. By understanding the role of nutrition in weight loss, individuals can create a diet plan that will help them reach their goals in a healthy and sustainable way. Nutrition plays a critical role in weight loss. Eating a healthy, balanced diet can help you reach and maintain a healthy weight, reduce your risk of chronic diseases, and improve your overall health. To lose weight and keep it off, you need to make sure that your diet provides enough energy (calories) to support your daily activities while helping you to achieve a caloric deficit. This means that you need to consume fewer calories than you burn.

The type of food you eat is also important. Eating nutrient-dense foods that are rich in vitamins, minerals, protein, fiber, and healthy fats can help you feel full for longer and promote weight loss. Avoiding processed foods, refined carbohydrates, and added sugars can also help you to lose weight.

In addition, drinking plenty of water throughout the day can help you to feel fuller and curb cravings. Eating regular meals and snacks can also help you to maintain energy levels and stay on track with your weight loss goals.

Finally, getting regular physical activity is another important step in the weight loss process. Eating a healthy diet and exercising regularly can help you to reach and maintain a healthy weight. Regular physical activity can also help to reduce stress, improve your mood, and boost your overall health.

## EATING FOR WEIGHT LOSS

Eating for weight loss is all about finding a balance between healthy nutrition and calorie control. To achieve a healthy weight loss, it is important to make small, achievable changes to your diet and lifestyle. Start by making sure that your meals are balanced with proteins, carbohydrates and healthy fats. This will help you to stay full for longer and prevent unhealthy cravings. It is also important to pay attention to portion sizes, as overeating can lead to weight gain.

The major healthy food that enhance Weight Loss:

**Lean Proteins:** Foods like chicken, fish, lean beef, eggs, and tofu are rich in proteins and can help you feel fuller for longer. Protein also helps your body burn more calories.

**Fruits and Vegetables:** Eating a diet rich in fruits and vegetables can help you lose weight and keep it off. Fruits and vegetables are high in fiber, which helps you feel full for longer and keeps your digestive system healthy.

**Whole Grains:** Whole grains like oats, brown rice, and quinoa are packed with nutrients and fiber. Eating whole grains can help you feel fuller for longer and can help with weight loss.

**Legumes:** Legumes like beans, lentils, and chickpeas are a great source of protein and fiber. Eating legumes can help you feel fuller for longer and can help with weight loss.

**Healthy Fats:** Foods like nuts, seeds, avocados, and olive oil are high in healthy fats and can help you feel fuller for longer. Eating healthy fats can also help you lose weight.

## HOW TO READ NUTRITION LABELS

**Serving Size:** Check the serving size and the number of servings to get an idea of how much of the product you should eat.

**Calories:** Check the number of calories per serving and compare it to other similar products.

**Nutrients:** Look at the nutrients listed on the nutrition label. These include vitamins, minerals, fats, carbohydrates, and proteins.

**Percent Daily Value (%DV):** This is the percent of each nutrient in one serving compared to the recommended daily amount. This helps you to make sure you're getting enough of the essential nutrients.

**Ingredients:** Check the ingredients list to make sure you're not allergic to any of the ingredients. It's also a good idea to check for any added sugars or unhealthy fats.

**Check for Nutrient Claims:** Look for any nutrient claims on the label. If the product has a high percentage of a certain nutrient, it will likely be highlighted on the packaging. You should always be wary of any nutrient claims that sound too good to be true.

# CHAPTER THREE

# DESIGNING A WEIGHT LOSS MEAL PLAN

Designing a weight loss meal plan is the process of creating a personalized nutrition plan to help a person achieve their weight loss goals. This involves taking into account their current physical activity level, dietary preferences, and health conditions to create meals that will provide adequate nutrition while helping them reach their desired weight. The meal plan should be designed around healthy, nutrient-dense foods, such as fruits, vegetables, lean proteins, whole grains, and healthy fats. It should also include smaller portions, adequate hydration, and regular physical activity to maximize results. Additionally, the meal plan should be tailored to the individual's needs and preferences to ensure sustainability and success.

## TIPS TO DESIGNING A WEIGHT LOSS MEAL PLAN FOR WOMEN

**Consult with A Nutritionist or Dietitian:** A nutritionist or dietitian can provide valuable insight into your eating habits and help you create a meal plan tailored to your individual needs.

**Determine Your Calorie Needs:** Calculate your Basal Metabolic Rate (BMR) to determine how many calories your body needs to maintain its weight, then subtract

500-1000 calories to create a calorie deficit for weight loss.

**Plan Meals and Snacks.** Make sure to plan meals and snacks that include a balance of protein, complex carbohydrates, and healthy fats. Eating smaller, more frequent meals can help you feel full and keep your metabolism running.

**Choose Nutrient-Dense Foods:** Foods like fruits, vegetables, beans, whole grains, and lean proteins are more nutritionally dense and contain fewer calories than processed foods.

**Monitor Portion Sizes:** Use measuring cups and spoons to ensure you are eating appropriate portion sizes.

**Stay Hydrated:** Drinking plenty of water helps you feel full and can help reduce cravings.

**Track Your Progress:** Keeping track of your progress will help you stay motivated and make adjustments as needed.

## HOW TO COMBINE DIFFERENT TYPES OF MACRO NUTRIENTS TO OPTIMIZE WEIGHT LOSS FOR WOMEN

Weight loss for women should include a balanced combination of macro nutrients including carbohydrates, fats, and proteins.

**Carbohydrates:** Women should focus on consuming complex carbohydrates which provide sustained energy. These include whole grains, quinoa, oats, beans, and lentils. Aim to consume at least 40% of your daily caloric intake from carbohydrates.

**Fats:** Healthy fats like omega-3 fatty acids, monounsaturated fats, and polyunsaturated fats should be a part of your diet. These provide essential fatty acids, help to reduce cholesterol levels, and can help to keep you full for longer. Aim for approximately 20-30% of your daily caloric intake from fats.

**Proteins:** Protein helps to build and maintain muscle mass. Women should aim to consume lean proteins like fish, poultry, eggs, and tofu. Aim for approximately 30-40% of your daily caloric intake from proteins.

Combining these three macro nutrients in the right proportions can help optimize weight loss for women. Eating a variety of whole, unprocessed foods including fruits, vegetables, whole grains, legumes, and lean proteins can help you reach your weight-loss goals.

## MEAL PLAN TIME- TABLE FOR WEIGHT LOSS IN WOMEN

MONDAY

Breakfast: Oatmeal with blueberries, banana, and almonds

Snack: Greek yogurt with almonds

Lunch: Grilled salmon with quinoa and steamed broccoli

Snack: Celery sticks with hummus

Dinner: Grilled chicken with brown rice and a side salad

TUESDAY

Breakfast: Scrambled egg whites with spinach and mushrooms

Snack: Apple slices with almond butter

Lunch: Tuna salad with celery and whole grain crackers

Snack: Cucumber slices with cottage cheese

Dinner: Grilled shrimp with quinoa and steamed asparagus

WEDNESDAY

Breakfast: Smoothie with banana, almond milk, and protein powder

Snack: Hard-boiled egg

Lunch: Vegetable soup with lentils and whole-grain bread

Snack: Carrots with hummus

Dinner: Baked salmon with steamed vegetables and brown rice

## THURSDAY

Breakfast: Omelet with spinach, mushrooms and feta cheese

Snack: Almonds

Lunch: Grilled chicken with quinoa and roasted vegetables

Snack: Apple slices with peanut butter

Dinner: Baked tilapia with roasted potatoes and a side salad

## FRIDAY

Breakfast: Avocado toast with egg whites

Snack: Greek yogurt with berries

Lunch: Tuna salad with whole grain crackers

Snack: Celery sticks with almond butter

Dinner: Grilled steak with sweet potatoes and steamed broccoli

## SATURDAY

Breakfast: Smoothie with banana, almond milk, and protein powder

Snack: Hard-boiled egg

Lunch: Vegetable wrap with hummus and whole grain wrap

Snack: Carrots with cottage cheese

Dinner: Baked salmon with quinoa and steamed asparagus

## SUNDAY

Breakfast: Oatmeal with blueberries, banana, and almonds

Snack: Greek yogurt with almonds

Lunch: Grilled chicken with brown rice and a side salad

Snack: Celery sticks with hummus

Dinner: Grilled shrimp with quinoa and steamed vegetables

# ALTERNATIVE MEAL PLAN RECIPE WITH INGREDIENTS, INSTRUCTIONS AND PREP TIME

Day 1:

Breakfast:

Overnight Oats

Ingredients:

-1/2 cup rolled oats

-1/2 cup almond milk

-1 tsp chia seeds

-1/4 tsp ground cinnamon

-1/4 cup blueberries

-1 Tbsp almond butter

-1 tsp honey

Instructions:

1. In a bowl, mix together the oats, almond milk, chia seeds, and ground cinnamon.

2. Place the mixture in an airtight container and refrigerate overnight.

3. In the morning, stir in the blueberries, almond butter, and honey.

4. Serve cold or heat in the microwave for 1-2 minutes.

Time: 5 minutes

Lunch:

Quinoa and Roasted Veggie Bowl

Ingredients:

-1 cup cooked quinoa

-1 cup diced sweet potato

-1 cup diced zucchini

-1/2 cup diced red peppers

-1/2 cup diced red onion

-2 cloves of garlic, minced

-2 tsp olive oil

-1/4 tsp sea salt

Instructions:

1. Preheat oven to 400 degrees F.

2. Line a baking sheet with parchment paper.

3. Place sweet potato, zucchini, red peppers, red onion, and garlic on the baking sheet.

4. Drizzle with olive oil and sprinkle with sea salt.

5. Roast for 25-30 minutes, or until vegetables are cooked through.

6. Serve roasted vegetables over cooked quinoa.

Prep Time: 10 minutes

Dinner:

Grilled Salmon with Asparagus

Ingredients:

-4 4-oz. salmon fillets

-1 tsp olive oil

-1/2 tsp garlic powder

-1/4 tsp sea salt

-1/4 tsp black pepper

-1 lb. asparagus, trimmed

Instructions:

1. Preheat grill to medium-high heat.

2. Brush salmon fillets with olive oil, and season with garlic powder, sea salt, and pepper.

3. Place salmon fillets and asparagus on the grill.

4. Grill salmon for 5-7 minutes per side, or until cooked through.

5. Grill asparagus for 8-10 minutes, or until tender-crisp.

6. Serve salmon and asparagus together.

Prep Time: 10 minutes

Day 2:

Breakfast:

Avocado Toast

Ingredients:

-2 slices whole wheat bread

-1/2 avocado, mashed

-1/4 tsp garlic powder

-1/4 tsp sea salt

-1/4 tsp black pepper

-1/4 cup cherry tomatoes, halved

Instructions:

1. Toast bread in a toaster.

2. In a small bowl, mash together avocado, garlic powder, sea salt, and black pepper.

3. Spread avocado mixture onto each slice of toast.

4. Top with cherry tomatoes.

5. Serve immediately.

Prep Time: 5 minutes

Lunch:

Tuna Salad Wrap

Ingredients:

-2 6-oz. cans of tuna, drained

-1/4 cup diced celery

-1 Tbsp diced red onion

-1 Tbsp plain Greek yogurt

-1 Tbsp mayonnaise

-1/4 tsp sea salt

-1/4 tsp black pepper

-2 whole wheat wraps

Instructions:

1. In a bowl, mix together tuna, celery, red onion, Greek yogurt, mayonnaise, sea salt, and black pepper.

2. Spread tuna mixture onto each wrap.

3. Roll up wraps and cut in half.

4. Serve immediately.

Prep Time: 10 minutes

Dinner:

Baked Chicken with Broccoli

Ingredients:

- 4 4-oz. boneless skinless chicken breasts

- 2 tsp olive oil

- 1/2 tsp garlic powder

- 1/4 tsp sea salt

- 1/4 tsp black pepper

- 2 cups broccoli florets

Instructions:

1. Preheat oven to 400 degrees F.

2. Line a baking sheet with parchment paper.

3. Place chicken breasts on the baking sheet.

4. Drizzle with olive oil, and season with garlic powder, sea salt, and pepper.

5. Place broccoli florets around the chicken.

6. Bake for 25-30 minutes, or until chicken is cooked through.

7. Serve chicken and broccoli together.

Prep Time: 10 minutes

Day 3:

Breakfast:

Fruit Smoothie

Ingredients:

-1/2 cup frozen banana slices

-1/2 cup frozen strawberries

-1/2 cup almond milk

-1/4 cup plain Greek yogurt

-1 Tbsp honey

Instructions:

1. Place all ingredients in a blender.

2. Blend until smooth.

3. Serve immediately.

Prep Time: 5 minutes

Lunch:

Turkey and Hummus Wrap

Ingredients:

-2 whole wheat wraps

-4 oz. sliced turkey

-1/4 cup cucumber slices

-1/4 cup red pepper slices

-1/4 cup hummus

Instructions:

1. Spread hummus onto each wrap.

2. Top with turkey, cucumber, and red pepper slices.

3. Roll up wraps and cut in half.

4. Serve immediately.

Prep Time: 10 minutes

Dinner:

Vegetable Stir-Fry

Ingredients:

-1 Tbsp olive oil

-1/2 cup diced onion

-1 cup diced carrots

-1 cup diced zucchini

-1 cup diced bell peppers

-1/4 cup vegetable broth

-1 tsp garlic powder

-1/4 tsp sea salt

-1/4 tsp black pepper

Instructions:

1. Heat olive oil in a large skillet over medium heat.

2. Add onion, carrots, zucchini, and bell peppers.

3. Cook for 5 minutes, or until vegetables are tender.

4. Add vegetable broth, garlic powder, sea salt, and black pepper.

5. Cook for an additional 5 minutes, or until vegetables are cooked through.

6. Serve warm.

Prep Time: 10 minutes

Day 4:

Breakfast:

Yogurt Parfait

Ingredients:

-1 cup plain Greek yogurt

-1/2 cup blueberries

-1/4 cup slivered almonds

-1/4 cup granola

Instructions:

1. Layer yogurt, blueberries, almonds, and granola in a bowl.

2. Serve immediately.

Prep Time: 5 minutes

Lunch:

Salad with Avocado

Ingredients:

-2 cups baby spinach

-1/2 cup diced tomatoes

-1/4 cup diced red onion

-1/4 cup black beans

-1/4 avocado, diced

- 1 Tbsp olive oil

- 1 Tbsp white wine vinegar

- 1/4 tsp sea salt

- 1/4 tsp black pepper

Instructions:

1. In a bowl, mix together spinach, tomatoes, red onion, black beans, and avocado.

2. Drizzle with olive oil and vinegar.

3. Sprinkle with sea salt and black pepper.

4. Toss to combine.

5. Serve immediately.

Prep Time: 10 minutes

Dinner:

Roasted Chickpeas

Ingredients:

-1 can chickpeas, drained and rinsed

-2 tsp olive oil

-1/2 tsp garlic powder

-1/4 tsp sea salt

-1/4 tsp black pepper

Instructions:

1. Preheat oven to 375 degrees F.

2. Line a baking sheet with parchment paper.

3. Place chickpeas on the baking sheet.

4. Drizzle with olive oil, and season with garlic powder, sea salt, and black pepper.

5. Bake for 25 minutes, or until crispy.

6. Serve warm.

Prep Time: 10 minutes

Day 5:

Breakfast:

Egg and Spinach Muffins

Ingredients:

-6 eggs

-1/2 cup cooked spinach, chopped

-1/4 cup diced red pepper

-1/4 cup diced red onion

-1/4 tsp sea salt

-1/4 tsp black pepper

Instructions:

1. Preheat oven to 375 degrees F.

2. Grease a muffin tin with cooking spray.

3. In a bowl, whisk together eggs, spinach, red pepper, red onion, sea salt, and black pepper.

4. Divide mixture evenly among the muffin tins.

5. Bake for 20-25 minutes, or until eggs are cooked through.

6. Serve warm.

Prep Time: 10 minutes

Lunch:

Black Bean Burrito Bowl

Ingredients:

- 1 cup cooked brown rice
- 1/2 cup black beans
- 1/4 cup diced tomatoes
- 1/4 cup diced red onion
- 1/4 cup corn
- 1/4 avocado, diced
- 1 Tbsp cilantro, chopped
- 1 tsp olive oil
- 1/4 tsp sea salt
- 1/4 tsp black pepper

Instructions:

1. In a bowl, mix together brown rice, black beans, tomatoes, red onion, corn, avocado, cilantro, olive oil, sea salt, and black pepper.

2. Serve warm.

Prep Time: 10 minutes

Dinner:

Baked Cod with Broccoli

Ingredients:

-4 4-oz. cod fillets

-2 tsp olive oil

-1/2 tsp garlic powder

-1/4 tsp sea salt

-1/4 tsp black pepper

-2 cups broccoli florets

Instructions:

1. Preheat oven to 400 degrees F.

2. Line a baking sheet with parchment paper.

3. Place cod fillets on the baking sheet.

4. Drizzle with olive oil, and season with garlic powder, sea salt, and black pepper.

5. Place broccoli florets around the cod.

6. Bake for 25-30 minutes, or until cod is cooked through.

7. Serve cod and broccoli together.

Prep Time: 10 minutes

Day 6:

Breakfast:

Oatmeal with Fruit

Ingredients:

- 1/2 cup rolled oats

- 1 cup almond milk

- 1/2 cup diced banana

- 1/4 cup blueberries

- 1 Tbsp walnuts, chopped

Instructions:

1. In a saucepan, bring almond milk to a boil.

2. Stir in oats and reduce heat to low.

3. Simmer for 5 minutes, or until oats are cooked through.

4. Stir in banana, blueberries, and walnuts.

5. Serve warm.

Prep Time: 10 minutes

Lunch:

Taco Salad

Ingredients:

- 2 cups baby spinach
- 1/2 cup cooked black beans
- 1/4 cup corn
- 1/4 cup diced tomatoes
- 1/4 cup diced red onion
- 1/4 cup diced avocado
- 1 Tbsp olive oil
- 1 Tbsp lime juice
- 1/4 tsp sea salt

-1/4 tsp black pepper

Instructions:

1. In a bowl, mix together spinach, black beans, corn, tomatoes, red onion, and avocado.

2. Drizzle with olive oil and lime juice.

3. Sprinkle with sea salt and black pepper.

4. Toss to combine.

5. Serve immediately.

Prep Time: 10 minutes

Dinner:

Grilled Chicken and Vegetables

Ingredients:

-4 4-oz. boneless skinless chicken breasts

- 2 tsp olive oil

- 1/2 tsp garlic powder

- 1/4 tsp sea salt

- 1/4 tsp black pepper

- 1 cup diced zucchini

- 1 cup diced bell peppers

Instructions:

1. Preheat grill to medium-high heat.

2. Brush chicken breasts with olive oil, and season with garlic powder, sea salt, and pepper.

3. Place chicken breasts and vegetables on the grill.

4. Grill chicken for 5-7 minutes per side, or until cooked through.

5. Grill vegetables for 8-10 minutes, or until tender-crisp.

6. Serve chicken and vegetables together.

Prep Time: 10 minutes

Day 7:

Breakfast:

Chia Seed Pudding

Ingredients:

-1/2 cup chia seeds

-1 cup almond milk

-1/4 tsp ground cinnamon

-1/4 cup diced mango

-1 Tbsp walnuts, chopped

-1 tsp honey

Instructions:

1. In a bowl, mix together chia seeds, almond milk, and ground cinnamon.

2. Place the mixture in an airtight container and refrigerate overnight.

3. In the morning, stir in the mango, walnuts, and honey.

4. Serve cold.

Prep Time: 5 minutes

Lunch:

Grilled Salmon Salad

Ingredients:

- 4 4-oz. salmon fillets

- 2 tsp olive oil

- 1/2 tsp garlic powder

- 1/4 tsp sea salt

- 1/4 tsp black pepper

- 2 cups baby spinach

- 1/4 cup diced tomatoes

- 1/4 cup diced red onion

- 1/4 cup diced cucumber

Instructions:

1. Preheat grill to medium-high heat.

2. Brush salmon fillets with olive oil, and season with garlic powder, sea salt, and pepper.

3. Place salmon fillets on the grill.

4. Grill for 5-7 minutes per side, or until cooked through.

5. In a bowl, mix together spinach, tomatoes, red onion, and cucumber.

6. Serve salmon and salad together.

Prep Time: 10 minutes

Dinner:

Stuffed Peppers

Ingredients:

-4 bell peppers, halved and seeded

-1 cup cooked quinoa

-1/2 cup diced tomatoes

-1/2 cup diced zucchini

-1/4 cup diced red onion

-1/4 cup black beans

-1 Tbsp olive oil

-1/4 tsp sea salt

-1/4 tsp black pepper

Instructions:

1. Preheat oven to 400 degrees F.

2. Line a baking sheet with parchment paper.

3. Place bell peppers on the baking sheet.

4. In a bowl, mix together quinoa, tomatoes, zucchini, red onion, black beans, olive oil, sea salt, and black pepper.

5. Divide mixture evenly among the bell pepper halves.

6. Bake for 25-30 minutes, or until peppers are tender.

7. Serve warm.

Prep Time: 10 minutes

# CHAPTER FOUR

# MAKING HEALTHY EATING HABIT STICK FOR WEIGHT LOSS.

Making healthy eating habits stick for weight loss requires a combination of dedication, planning and hard work. Here are are a few hints to assist you with accomplishing your weight - loss objectives

**Prepare Meals Ahead Of Time:** When you plan your meals ahead of time, you make it easier to stick to healthy eating habits. Meal prepping can help reduce the temptation to reach for unhealthy snacks.

**Set Realistic Goals:** Setting achievable goals will help you stay motivated and on track. Choose a goal that is reasonable and achievable.

**Make Healthy Swaps:** Instead of reaching for chips, try swapping them out for air-popped popcorn or a few slices of an apple with a tablespoon of nut butter. Choose healthier versions of your favorite foods, such as whole-grain bread or quinoa instead of white bread.

**Track Your Progress:** Tracking your progress can help keep you motivated and on track with your weight-loss goals. Use an app or journal to record your meals and snacks.

**Get Enough Sleep:** Lack of sleep can lead to increased hunger and cravings for unhealthy foods. Aim for 7-9 hours of sleep each night.

**Stay Hydrated:** Staying hydrated can help keep your hunger levels in check and help you avoid overeating. Aim to drink at least 8 glasses of water per day.

**Move Your Body:** Exercise is an important part of any weight loss plan. Aim for at least 30 minutes of exercise per day.

By following these tips, you can make healthy eating habits stick for weight loss and reach your goals.

# CHAPTER FIVE

# AVOIDING COMMON DIET PITFALLS

Avoiding Common Diet Pitfalls for Weight Loss means avoiding bad habits and mistakes that can lead to unhealthy eating patterns and ultimately impede weight loss. Examples of these common diet pitfalls include skipping meals, relying on pre-packaged and processed foods, not eating enough fruits and vegetables, overeating, becoming too restrictive with food choices, and

pursuing extreme diets. To avoid these pitfalls, it is important to:

1. Plan Your Meals Ahead of Time: Planning out your meals for the week will help you stay on track and avoid unhealthy meals. Preparing healthy meals ahead of time will also save you time in the long run.

2. Don't Skip Meals: Skipping meals can cause you to overeat later in the day, leading to unhealthy food choices. Eating regular meals throughout the day will help keep your metabolism going, while also preventing hunger-driven cravings.

3. Avoid Processed Foods: Processed foods are packed with unhealthy additives, sodium, and preservatives, making them a poor choice for anyone looking to maintain a healthy diet.

Eating fresh, whole foods will ensure you're getting the nutrients you need to stay healthy.

4. Drink Plenty of Water: Drinking plenty of water will help you stay full and hydrated, while also flushing toxins out of your system. Water is essential for good health, so try to avoid sugary drinks and stick to plain old H2O.

5. Don't Get Too Restrictive: It's important to be mindful of what you're eating, but overly restrictive diets can often lead to unhealthy behaviors, such as binging or obsessing over food. It's important to find a balance that works for you and allows you to enjoy your meals.

# CHAPTER SIX

# INCORPORATING EXERCISE INTO YOUR WEIGHT LOSS PLAN

Exercise is a vital part of any weight loss plan. Not only does it help you burn calories and fat, but regular physical activity also increases your metabolism, improves your overall health, boosts your mood, and helps you maintain your weight loss.

When creating a weight loss plan, it's important to choose exercises that you enjoy and are realistic for your lifestyle. Aim to include at least 30 minutes of exercise each day. Start with low-intensity activities such as walking, swimming, or biking, and gradually increase your intensity as your fitness level improves.

Exercising regularly can be a great way to improve your overall health and wellbeing. Making exercise a part of your daily life is a great way to stay motivated and healthy. Here are some tips to help you make exercise a part of your daily life:

**Start Small:** Don't try to do too much too soon. Start with something that is manageable and gradually increase the intensity or duration as you become more fit.

**Make A Plan:** Write down a schedule of when and how you will exercise, and make sure to stick to it.

**Find An Activity You Enjoy:** Exercise doesn't have to be boring or mundane. Find an activity that you enjoy doing, whether it be running, swimming, biking, or something else.

**Set Goals:** Make realistic goals for yourself and track your progress. This will help to keep you motivated.

**Make Time for Yourself:** Exercise can be a great way to de-stress and take some time for yourself. Set aside some time each day to focus on your physical health.

**Find an accountability partner:** Having an accountability partner can help to keep you on track and motivated.

Making exercise a part of your daily life is a great way to stay healthy and look and feel your best. With a bit of planning and dedication, you can make exercise a habit and reap the rewards.

## TYPES OF EXERCISES FOR WEIGHT LOSS IN WOMEN

Weight loss exercises for women should include both cardio and strength training. To lose weight and keep it off, women should aim for at least 150 minutes of moderate-intensity cardio each week. Examples of moderate-intensity activities include walking, jogging, and biking.

**Strength training** is also important for weight loss. It helps build lean muscle mass and boost your metabolism. Aim to do 2–3 strength training workouts each week, focusing on your major muscle groups. Examples of strength training exercises include squats, lunges, push-ups, and weight lifting.

**Interval training** is also a great way to get your heart pumping and burn calories. This type of exercise alternates between periods of high-intensity and low-intensity activity. It's a great way to get more out of your workouts in less time.

**Yoga and Pilates** are also great exercises for weight loss. They help build strength and flexibility, while also promoting mindfulness.

Finally, don't forget about **stretching.** It increases flexibility, which can help make your workouts more comfortable and effective. Stretches such as downward dog, cobra, and cat-cow are all great options.

Overall, to get the most out of your workouts, aim to incorporate a variety of cardio, strength training, interval training, yoga, Pilates, and stretching into your routine. With a little bit of effort, you'll be losing weight and feeling great in no time.

# CHAPTER SEVEN

# MAINTAINING YOUR WEIGHT LOSS

Maintaining your weight loss means making a commitment to healthy eating habits and regular physical activity for the long term. This means eating a balanced diet with a variety of nutrient-dense foods, monitoring caloric intake, and avoiding "crash" diets. Additionally, it means engaging in regular physical activity that includes aerobic and strength-training exercises. Lastly, it means staying motivated to continue with the changes you've made.

**Set Realistic Goals:** Losing weight and keeping it off requires long-term commitment and dedication. Set realistic goals for yourself and be sure to set smaller milestones that will help you reach your overall goal.

**Track Your Progress:** Tracking your progress can help motivate you and keep you on track. Use a food journal, fitness tracker, or tracking app to help you monitor your progress and how you're doing.

**Eat Healthy:** Eating healthy is key to maintaining your weight loss. Choose nutrient-dense foods such as lean proteins, fruits, vegetables, whole grains, and healthy fats.

**Exercise regularly:** Exercise is essential for maintaining weight loss. Aim for at least 30 minutes of moderate intensity activity per day.

**Stay Motivated:** Staying motivated is crucial to maintaining your weight loss. Find ways to stay motivated such as joining a gym, finding an online support group, or setting realistic goals with rewards.

**Manage Stress:** Stress can cause weight gain and prevent you from maintaining your weight loss. Try to

find healthy coping mechanisms such as yoga, meditation, or talking to a friend.

**Get Enough Sleep:** Getting enough sleep is important for weight loss and maintenance. Aim for 7-9 hours of sleep per night to ensure your body is well rested.

**Avoid Temptation:** Avoid temptation by avoiding places or situations that may trigger unhealthy eating habits.

**Be Consistent:** Consistency is key to maintaining your weight loss. Stick to your healthy eating and exercise habits and don't let yourself get off track.

## CONCLUSION:

In conclusion, the Weight Loss Diet Book for Women is an invaluable resource for any woman looking to achieve her weight loss goals. It provides a comprehensive overview of the most popular diet plans and strategies for weight loss, as well as tips and tricks for making weight loss easier and more enjoyable. It also offers a wealth of information on nutrition, exercise, and lifestyle changes that can help women achieve their weight loss goals. With the help of this book, women can learn about various diet plans, find the one that best suits their needs, and make the necessary changes to their lifestyle to see real results. Ultimately, this book provides the necessary information and support to help women reach their desired weight safely and effectively.